Copyright © 2021

All rights reserved. No part of this publication maybe reproduced, distributed, or transmitted in any form or by any means, including photocopying, recording, or other electronic or mechanical methods, without the prior written permission of the publisher, except in the case of brief quotations embodied in critical reviews and certain other noncommercial uses permitted by copyright law.

Contents

What is Nutrisystem Diet?

Nutrisystem is a commercial weight-loss diet that involves eating the company's prepackaged and delivered meals and snacks, along with some produce you shop for yourself. The program boasts that it can help you lose up to 18 pounds (8 kg) in 2 months, and some people have reported weight loss success from the diet.

Nutrisystem is also built around the glycemic index, a measure of how various carbs affect your blood sugar. The program is high in protein and emphasizes "good" carbs, such as many veggies and whole grains that are digested slowly. That keeps you feeling full longer and your blood sugar and metabolism from going out of whack. Depending on your plan – there are gender-specific tracks for adults, vegetarians and people living with diabetes – you'll eat five to six times a day. The program can also be customized for those needing a lower sodium (about 1,500 mg/day) level.

What is the Nutrisystem diet plan?

The Nutrisystem diet plan consists of eating several smaller meals each day.

Though their plans vary based on a person's preferences and cost, some common features include:

• 7-days worth of meals

• breakfast, lunch, dinner, and three snacks throughout the day

• frozen and fresh meals, shakes, and nutritional guides

- NuMi Weight Loss App (Uniquely Yours and Uniquely Yours Ultimate)
- unlimited support

According to Nutrisystem, eating smaller, balanced meals six times a day helps prevent hunger and promotes weight loss. However, some studies contradict this theory.

In an older study, researchers found that increasing meals from three to six a day did not impact a person's body's ability to burn fat.

Contrary to Nutrisystem's claims, the researchers found that increased meal frequency might lead to increased hunger and a desire to eat.

A more recent study from 2017 had similar results. In this study, researchers found that decreasing meal frequency throughout the day, and having the largest meal in the morning helped prevent long-term weight gain.

How Nutrisystem works

Method

Nutrisystem is a 4-week program. However, you can repeat the 4-week program as many times as you would like.

On Nutrisystem, you should aim to eat six small meals per day — breakfast, lunch, dinner, and three snacks. Several of these will be frozen meals or shakes provided by Nutrisystem.

Week 1 is a little bit different from the remainder of the program. During this week, you eat three meals, one snack, and one specially formulated Nutrisystem shake per day. This supposedly prepares your body for weight loss success.

However, during the remaining 3 weeks, you should aim to eat six times per day. For meals and snacks that are not provided by Nutrisystem, the company recommends choosing lean, low calorie, and low sodium options.

Each week, you're also allowed a total of up to eight "Flex Meals" — two breakfasts, two lunches, two dinners, and two snacks — to account for meals that may not be ideal for weight loss but may be part of a holiday or special occasion.

You can also use the free NuMi app provided by Nutrisystem for meal planning guidance.

Specialized programs

Nutrisystem offers several meal plans to cater to different dietary needs. In addition, each meal plan features the following pricing tiers:

- Basic: least expensive, provides 5 days of food each week
- Uniquely Yours: most popular, provides 5 days of food each week along with customization options
- Ultimate: most expensive, provides 7 days of food each week along with customization options

You can also select your own meal plan. The meal plans offered by Nutrisystem include:

- Standard: The standard Nutrisystem plan is targeted toward women and contains a variety of popular meals and snacks.

- Men's: Nutrisystem Men's contains additional snacks each week and includes meals that are more appealing to most men.

- Nutrisystem D: Nutrisystem D is for people who have type 2 diabetes. These meals are high in protein and fiber, with a focus on foods that will not cause rapid blood sugar spikes.

- Vegetarian: This meal plan contains no meat but features dairy products — so it's not appropriate for vegans.

Can Nutrisystem help you lose weight?

Nutrisystem — like most diet plans — may aid short-term weight loss.

If the diet is followed closely, your daily calorie intake will average 1,200–1,500 calories — which, for most people, is a calorie deficit that will result in weight loss.

The Nutrisystem website states that you can expect to lose 1–2 pounds (0.5–1 kg) per week if you follow the diet, but that you can lose up to 18 pounds (8 kg) "fast."

This finding was based on the results of a study that was funded by Nutrisystem and not published in a peer-reviewed scientific journal.

In this study in 84 adults, those on Nutrisystem lost twice as much weight as people on the Dietary Approaches to Stop Hypertension (DASH) diet after 4 weeks.

The same study found that the average weight loss after 12 weeks on Nutrisystem was 18 pounds (8 kg).

One study in 69 adults with type 2 diabetes found that those following Nutrisystem lost significantly more weight in 3 months than those in a control group who received diabetes education but no specialized diet program.

Still, research on long-term weight maintenance after doing Nutrisystem is lacking.

Does Nutrisystem Diet have any health risks?

No indications of serious short-term risks or side effects on Nutrisystem have surfaced. But the company does not recommend its program for people with certain health conditions or dietary restrictions. Among them:

• Pregnant women, who generally require additional calories, should not follow Nutrisystem.

• Women breastfeeding an infant who is younger than 6 months or who has not yet begun solid foods, also aren't appropriate Nutrisystem dieters, though there's a higher-calorie Nutrisystem plan for lactating women.

- Anyone under 18 should not be on Nutrisystem, since children and teenagers are still growing.

- The Nutrisystem Diet won't suit people with peanut or soy allergies, since these ingredients are commonly found in Nutrisystem meals.

Is Nutrisystem Diet a heart-healthy diet?

Nutrisystem is probably a good diet for heart health. The 2013 study in the American Journal of Hypertension found that, in addition to weight and fat loss, participants on Nutrisystem's plan significantly reduced their blood pressure and arterial stiffness.

Other company data shows decreased blood pressure, total and bad LDL cholesterol levels, and triglycerides, a fatty substance that in excess has been linked to heart disease, for some dieters on the program. If you're overweight or obese and shed some pounds on Nutrisystem, you'll undoubtedly do your heart a favor – weight loss is commonly associated with decreased blood pressure, cholesterol and risk of heart disease.

Can Nutrisystem Diet prevent or control diabetes?

Nutrisystem may help prevent or control diabetes.

Prevention: Excess weight is a major cause of Type 2 diabetes, so if Nutrisystem's packaged meals and portion control help you shed pounds and keep them off, you'll stand a better chance of avoiding the chronic disease. Unpublished research on over 32,000 Nutrisystem customers who tracked their weights for six months showed that 86% lost at least 5% of their weight, and 63% lost at least 10% of their weight. Company-funded research has also shown Nutrisystem helps lower fasting blood glucose levels. In a 2016 study in the journal Obesity Reviews, researchers compared the glycemic benefits of three commercial diet plans including Nutrisystem among overweight and obese participants in 18 randomized trials, most of whom did not have Type 2 diabetes. While Jenny Craig reduced A1C levels most among all participants, Nutrisystem also significantly reduced A1C levels more than counseling at six months.

Control: Nutrisystem's diabetes program, Nutrisystem D, differs only slightly from its mainstream adult plans – both provide about the same number of calories and similar amounts of fat, protein and carbs. Dieters on Nutrisystem D have fewer menu options (higher-GI and higher-sugar foods are excluded) and may be on a different eating schedule. The "D" program helped dieters lower their fasting blood sugar and hemoglobin A1C levels – a measure of blood sugar over time – according to the two studies detailed in the "Will you lose weight?" section.

The 2013 study found that obese diabetics on the company's "D" program reduced their A1C significantly more than dieters assigned to diabetes self-management education. The study also found that 72% of the Nutrisystem group met the American Diabetes Association goal of tight blood sugar control – an A1C level of less than 7% – at six months, compared with only 44% of the control group. What's more, 28% of Nutrisystem dieters reduced the intensity of their diabetes medication regimen at the six-month mark, while only 4% of control dieters did.

Those results challenge an earlier, small study showing that, after six months, diabetics on Nutrisystem's "D" program reduced their A1C levels more than control dieters did, but the difference was not significant. Based on a few trials that included people with Type 2 diabetes in the 2016 Obesity Reviews review, the researchers noted that "Nutrisystem significantly reduced A1c 0.3 percent more than counseling at 6 months."

Does Nutrisystem Diet allow for restrictions and preferences?

Not everyone will be able to customize Nutrisystem to their needs – choose your preference for more information.

Is a supplement recommended? Yes, Nutrisystem endorses multivitamins for all dieters.

Vegetarian or Vegan: Nutrisystem offers vegetarian plans (for those who consume dairy and eggs), including frozen options and 104 vegetarian foods. Nutrisystem, however, has no vegan plan.

Gluten-Free: There are too few gluten-free foods to offer a meal plan

Low-Salt: If you're willing to sacrifice a little variety – and crunch numbers – you can customize meal choices and grocery additions to be as low as 1,500 milligrams of sodium, according to the company.

Kosher: There is no Nutrisystem plan for kosher dieters.

Halal: Nutrisystem does not offer a plan for halal eaters.

What To Keep In Mind

The Nutrisystem daily plan allows for three meals plus one snack for women or two snacks for men. There is no specific meal timing and fasting is not required for the plan. There are no special books to buy but the NuMi app is strongly recommended. Weight-loss counselors are also available by phone.

Nutrisystem's counselors are not required to have a nutrition degree, although they will have either an associate's degree or a bachelor's degree. They are also encouraged to be knowledgeable in nutrition, fitness, health, and weight loss maintenance.

But Nutrisystem is not for everyone. According to the company, women who are pregnant should not go on Nutrisystem since they need additional calories. If you are breastfeeding and your child is at least 6 months old and is eating solid foods, you can use a modified Nutrisystem plan that affords more calories. Nutrisystem provides a phone number to contact for more information.

Additionally, people who have celiac disease are not advised to use the Nutrisystem diet, according to the website. They offer a few menu items that do not include gluten ingredients and can offer a wheat-free menu, but they do not offer certified gluten-free foods.

Other people who should not use Nutrisystem including anyone who is allergic to soy, peanuts, or latex, a person who has an eating disorder such as anorexia or bulimia, those with chronic kidney disease, or those following a ketogenic diet. Women weighing 400 pounds or more and men weighing 450 pounds or more require a doctor's approval prior to starting a Nutrisystem plan.

What To Eat?

Nutrisystem offers a tier of programs to suit various weight loss goals and different budgets. There are separate programs for men and women, as well as plans for vegetarians and people who have type 2 diabetes. Each plan provides three meals per day plus one snack for women and two snacks for men.

There are three plan levels ("Basic," "Uniquely Yours," and "Uniquely Yours Ultimate"), each offering slightly different choices for food. On each plan, you will receive portion-controlled meals as well as access to online tools and a smartphone app. Questions, concerns, and requests for general support are addressed by weight loss counselors who are available by phone.

Within each plan, you can choose your own meals or have meals selected for you ("Chef's Choice"). You can also personalize meal choices based on your body type, goals, and food preferences. To select this option, you will take a short automated quiz.

Most of the food that you eat on the plan is provided by Nutrisystem. "Basic" meals are shelf-stable (not frozen) but the higher quality meals in the "Uniquely Yours" and "Uniquely Yours Ultimate" plans include both frozen and non-frozen selections. The more expensive plans include a wider variety of options in terms of meal and snack choices.

The first week of the program is designed to "reboot your body," and it is more restrictive than subsequent weeks. During this week, you only consume the brand's food and shakes. This weeklong program is designed for quick weight loss of fewer than 10 pounds and can be purchased without investing in a longer-term meal plan.

After the first week, Nutrisystem customers incorporate two flex meals during the week. These meals are prepared using ingredients that you purchase. Grocery guides are provided so customers know what foods are compliant. Restaurant meals are allowed as flex meals. The NuMi app provides specific guidance for which menu items to select and which to avoid when dining out.

Foods to Eat

- Prepackaged meals and snacks from Nutrisystem
- Lean proteins (limited)
- Carbohydrates (limited)
- Some vegetables
- Some healthy fats
- Some condiments, seasonings, spices
- Some beverages (including alcohol)

Foods To Avoid

- Store-bought food other than those listed as compliant

- Sweets and desserts other than those listed as compliant

Prepackaged Meals and Snacks

Nutrisystem meals include comfort-food selections such as double chocolate muffins, macaroni and cheese, grilled chicken sandwiches, or pizza. Each provides around 200 calories. The bars also come in a variety of flavors such as apple strudel or toffee nut and contain about 200 calories each.

The system's shakes ("NutriCrush" or "Turbo Shakes") contain whey protein, flavors, sweeteners, and herbal ingredients such as monk fruit. Shakes provide around 120 calories per serving (without milk).

Lean Proteins

Nutrisystem provides a list of approved proteins, called "PowerFuels." Each serving is supposed to provide 5 grams of protein and 80–120 calories.

The list includes meat, seafood, poultry, plant-based protein, low-fat dairy, and nuts. Examples include 2 ounces of trimmed beef, 1 tablespoon of nut butter or tahini, 1/2 cup seitan, 2 ounces of canned salmon, 1 egg, or 1 cup of non-fat plain yogurt.

Carbohydrates

Nutrisystem provides a list of "SmartCarbs"—low glycemic carbs that provide fiber. Each serving is supposed to provide at least 1 gram of fiber and 80–120 calories.

The approved list includes whole grains, beans and legumes, fruit, and starchy vegetables. Examples include one medium banana, apple, or orange, 1/2 cup oatmeal, a 6-inch whole-wheat pita, 1/4 cup whole-grain crackers, or 1 cup of canned fruit cocktail.

Vegetables

Customers are strongly encouraged to consume at least 4 servings of non-starchy vegetables each day. You can also consume low-sodium vegetable juice as an alternative.

Each serving is equivalent to 1/2 cup cooked or 1 cup raw of approved veggies including bell peppers, broccoli, any kind of lettuce, green beans, cucumbers, asparagus, and tomatoes.

Condiments, Seasoning, Spices

Foods defined as "Extras" and "Free Foods" allow you to prepare, season, and flavor your food. Approved "Free-Food" seasonings should provide no more than 10 calories per serving but are unlimited on the plan. Free condiments include mustard, garlic, ginger, and salsa.

"Extras" should only provide 10–35 calories per serving. Ketchup, honey, and mayonnaise are considered extras. Some healthy fats like avocado and sunflower oil are also considered extras, but you'll need to limit your intake to stay within calorie limits.

Beverages

You can drink black coffee, unsweetened tea, herbal tea, and seltzer on the plan. You are also encouraged to drink at least 64 ounces of water each day.

Nutrisystem's Food Guide

Nutrisystem encourages lean, low calorie, and high fiber choices. Foods that are high in calories, fat, or both should be avoided on this diet.

While on Nutrisystem, the majority of your meals and snacks are provided for you.

On the basic plans, you'll receive four meals — breakfast, lunch, dinner, and one snack — for 5 days each week. As such, you'd need to add two snacks each day for 5 days, as well as all six meals for the remaining 2 days of each week.

On the "Ultimate" plans, you'll receive four meals for each day of the week, so you only need to provide two additional snacks each day.

Below are some guidelines regarding foods you should eat (in addition to the meals and snacks provided by Nutrisystem) and avoid on the diet.

How much should you exercise on Nutrisystem Diet?

Exercise is encouraged, but not required, on Nutrisystem. The program encourages dieters to engage in at least 30 minutes of physical activity each day, which can be broken up into three 10-minute intervals.

Nutrisystem offers some pointers to get you started. You can browse beginner, intermediate and advanced exercise programs online with detailed explanations of stretches and exercises. For extra motivation, you can log every pickup basketball game and bench press or read fitness tips on the website The Leaf.

Benefits and Drawbacks

Benefits

- Convenient
- Wide variety of foods
- Nutritionally balanced
- Transition plans offered
- Exercise is encouraged

Drawbacks

- Cost
- Processed foods

Benefits

Convenience

Proponents of the Nutrisystem plan find it easy to follow because foods are pre-portioned to keep calories low, which can promote weight loss. Having meals delivered to your door is a convenience factor that some people find appealing.

Variety

Flex meals, snacks, and supplementary foods can help to make the menu more varied, such as SmartCarbs, PowerFuels, Extras, and Free Foods. Easy-to-follow grocery lists help to simplify shopping.

Balanced

The plan provides between 1,200 to 1,500 calories per day and many foods contain protein, carbohydrate, fat, and nutrients such as fiber. Customers are encouraged to consume at least four servings of veggies and one to two servings of fruit each day, and support is offered to those who may find this challenging.

Transition Support

Exercise is encouraged and guidance is provided to help you start a program. Once you've reached your goal weight, a weight-maintenance plan is offered. These plans include weekend meal plans or a combination of meals and snacks. Of course, there is an additional fee for these products.

Drawbacks

Cost

Like many commercial weight loss plans, Nutrisystem won't fit into everyone's budget. The program can cost approximately $250 to $350 per month plus the cost of additional foods from the grocery store such as vegetables, fruit, and dairy that you'll need to supplement your diet.

Processed Foods

The prepackaged food on the Nutrisystem diet is heavily processed. You'll find plenty of unfamiliar ingredients in the meals and snacks. And if you are concerned about GMOs, the company is clear that their foods may contain them. Nutrisystem does not, however, use stimulants or appetite suppressants in its shakes and bars. Additionally, many of the low-calorie processed foods included in the diet tend to be high-calorie foods when purchased at restaurants or grocery stores.

Potential Health Benefits

Many people have had weight loss success on the Nutrisystem diet because it is a low-calorie eating plan. The entrées and snacks associated with the diet may also help those who follow the plan to learn portion control.

According to research published in the Annals of Internal Medicine in 2015, people who followed the Nutrisystem plan lost an average of 3.8% more weight over a three-month period than a control group who received nutritional counseling and education.

Potential Health Risks

While there are no common health risks associated with the Nutrisystem diet, the eating plan is centered on many frozen and processed pre-made foods that are not healthy food choices. Some foods on the Nutrisystem menu such as double chocolate muffins, frozen pizza bowls, and snickerdoodle cookies are not very nutritious.

This could make it harder for some people to choose healthy foods over processed foods once they end their subscription and resume a regular diet. Research shows that long-term consumption of processed foods is associated with chronic diseases.

Nutrisystem menu plans

Nutrisystem offers plans for people with health conditions and dietary preferences.

Diabetes

Nutrisystem offers a dietary option geared towards people living with diabetes. The diabetes option is also similar in price to their other dietary plans.

The diabetes plan includes meals and snacks that a person eats every 2–3 hours to help keep their blood sugar levels steady. The foods also aim to help a person feel fuller for longer.

According to Nutrisystem, their plans will help with:

- managing blood glucose levels

- weight loss

A 2009 study supports the use of dietary programs for helping people with diabetes. The researchers found that people living with obesity and type 2 diabetes saw improvements in weight, glucose control, and cardiovascular disease risk.

Obesity

Nutrisystem claims to help with weight loss, which can benefit people living with obesity. Some studies support these weight-loss claims. However, the long-term effects and sustainability of the program are still unclear and require further research.

Vegetarians

People following a vegetarian diet plan can still use Nutrisystem. The vegetarian plan is more expensive than the Basic plan, but not as expensive as their Ultimate plan.

Males

Nutrisystem offers specialized plans for males. The menu includes more snacks and more calories for males than the plans for females.

Alternative programs

There are other programs similar to Nutrisystem.

They include:

- JennyCraig
- WeightWatchers
- Atkins

- South Beach Diet

All dietary programs and menus are slightly different. A person should look for a program or plan that works best for their needs.

Before making dietary changes, a person should talk to their doctor or nutritionist, who can help them choose the best option based on their health and dietary needs.

Nutrisystem's Food List

In addition to the meals provided, here are the foods you can eat on Nutrisystem:

Proteins: lean meats, legumes, nuts, seeds, tofu, meat substitutes

Fruits: apples, oranges, bananas, strawberries, blueberries, blackberries, tomatoes, avocados

Vegetables: salad greens, spinach, kale, broccoli, cauliflower, carrots, cabbage, asparagus, mushrooms, turnips, radishes, onions

Fats: cooking spray, plant-based (lower calorie) spreads or oils

Dairy: skim or low fat milk, low fat yogurts, reduced-fat cheeses

Carbs: whole grain breads, whole grain pastas, sweet potatoes, brown rice, oats

Nutrisystem Sample meal plan

This 3-day sample menu outlines what the "basic" Nutrisystem plan may be like. Use this to help you with meal planning on your Nutrisystem diet. Nutrisystem typically provides 4 meals, 5 days per week, so this menu includes 2 days with Nutrisystem meals and 1 day with no Nutrisystem meals.

Day 1

- Breakfast: Nutrisystem Cranberry and Orange Muffin
- Snack 1: strawberries and low fat yogurt
- Lunch: Nutrisystem Hamburger
- Snack 2: celery and almond butter
- Dinner: Nutrisystem Chicken Pot Pie
- Snack 3: Nutrisystem S'mores Pie

Day 2

- Breakfast: Nutrisystem Biscotti Bites
- Snack 1: protein shake made with skim milk

- Lunch: Nutrisystem Spinach and Cheese Pretzel Melt
- Snack 2: baby carrots and hummus
- Dinner: Nutrisystem Cheesesteak Pizza
- Snack 3: Nutrisystem Ice Cream Sandwich

Day 3

- Breakfast: multigrain cereal with skim milk, banana
- Snack 1: apple and peanut butter
- Lunch: turkey and cheese sandwich on whole wheat bread
- Snack 2: whole grain crackers and cheese
- Dinner: baked salmon, brown rice, salad with vinaigrette dressing

Snack 3: 2–4 squares of dark chocolate

NUTRISYSTEM DIET RECIPES

Trying nutrisystem recipes is a great way to explore new flavors and find new favorite dishes while looking after your health. In this part are nourishing nutrisystem diet recipes for you to enjoy and lose weight fast.

Fettuccine Alfredo with Chicken

Prepartion time

30 minutes

INGREDIENTS

- 16 oz fettuccine

- 2 boneless, skinless chicken breasts
- 10 fresh sliced mushrooms (optional)
- 4 Tbsp butter, divided
- 2 Tbsp flour
- 1 tsp dried parsley
- 1/2 tsp onion powder
- 1/2 tsp salt
- 1/2 tsp pepper
- 2 cups 2% milk
- 1/2 c grated Parmesan cheese

Instructions

1. Prepare fettuccine according to directions; toss with 2 Tbsp butter.

2. Meanwhile, melt remaining butter (2 Tbsp) in large saute pan.

3. Add chicken, cut into bite-sized pieces (10 fresh, sliced mushrooms are a nice addition, too--not included in this calorie count).

4. Cook approximately 10 minutes or until chicken is done.

5. Stir in flour, parsley, onion powder, salt, and pepper.

6. Add milk; stir continuously while bringing it to a boil until mixture thickens slightly.

7. Add fettuccine and Parmesan cheese, tossing to coat.

8. Serve immediately. Makes approximately 10 (1 c) servings. Excellent with sides of salad, corn, and French bread!

Gallo Pinto (Costa Rican Black Beans & Rice)

Prepartion time

20 minutes

INGREDIENTS

- 2 cups Rice (pre-cooked/leftovers)
- 1 cup Black Beans (pre-cooked/leftovers)
- 2 cloves Garlic minced
- cup Onion diced
- cup Sweet Peppers diced
- cup Celery diced
- Cilantro
- Salsa Lizano
- Tabasco

Instructions

1. Saute garlic, onion, sweet peppers and celery in a large skillet.

2. Add beans (with a little of the bean broth) and stir until thoroughly heated.

3. Smash a few of the beans for a thicker consistency.

4. Add cooked rice and stir until thoroughly heated.

5. Add Salsa Lizano and Tabasco to taste and garnish with fresh chopped cilantro just before serving.

Cinnaproccino (Coffee Cinnamon Protein Shake)

Prepartion time

5 minutes

INGREDIENTS

- Cup of ice
- 1/2 c. of cold brewed coffee (I use leftover)
- 1/2 c. of skim milk
- 1 scoop vanilla whey protein powder
- 2 dropperfuls of liquid stevia - or - 1/4 tsp. powdered stevia
- Couple shakes of cinnamon

Instructions

1. In a blender, put a cup of ice.

2. Add coffee, milk, protein powder, stevia, and cinnamon. Blend to frothy shake. Makes approximately 1 - 12.oz shake.

3. Sprinkle cinnamon on top, grab a straw, and treat yourself.

MY healthy Chicken Sour Cream Enchilada's

Prepartion time

1 hour

INGREDIENTS

- 12oz. or about 3 chicken breasts
- 1c chopped onion
- Garlic powder to taste
- Red pepper to taste
- 10 corn tortillias
- 0.5c cream of chicken soup
- 0.25c sour cream
- 1c fat free chedder cheese
- cilantro
- 0.5c 1% milk

Instructions

1. boil chicken then shred into small peices, saute onion add to chicken season with garlic and pepper, Warm tortillias, Warm soup, sour cream and milk in sauce pan, fill tortillia's with chicken, sprinkle a little cheese and cilantro in each one.

2. Pour sour cream sauce on top of all enchilada's and sprinkle with remaining cheese.

3. Bake at 350 for 15 to 20 minutes.

Coffee Protein Breakfast Shake

Prepartion time

5 minutes

INGREDIENTS

- 2 cups brewed coffee
- 1 Cup Milk, (2% is used in the calorie count)
- 1 Scoop (2.95 tbsp) Protein Powder

Instructions

1. Put all ingredients into blender or blender cup, and blend or shake until smooth.

Chocolate Protein Shake

Prepartion time

5 minutes

INGREDIENTS

- 1/2 cup cottage cheese (non-fat or 1%)
- 1/2 cup milk (skim or 1%)
- 1 tbsp cocoa powder
- 1/2 tsp vanilla
- 2 packets splenda
- 5 ice cubes

Instructions

1. Combine all ingredients in blender until smooth. Enjoy!

Protein-Rich Chocolate Shake

Prepartion time

5 minutes

INGREDIENTS

- 1 packet Truvia sweetener
- 2 tsp. dark hot chocolate powder
- 1/4 cup cottage cheese, 2%
- 3/4 cup skim milk
- 1/4 tsp vanilla extract
- 4 ice cubes

Instructions

1. Combine all ingredients in a blender and blend until smooth. Enjoy!

Raw Chocolate Protein Shake

Prepartion time

5 minutes

INGREDIENTS

- 1 cup of almond milk
- 1 ripe banana, chopped, frozen
- 1 T. raw cocoa powder (2 T. if adding spinach)
- 1 scoop of protein powder

- vanilla 1 handful of organic baby spinach (optional)
- ice cubes

Instructions

1. Blend in blender container! Adjust measurements to suit your taste. Enjoy this raw chocolate protein shake recipe!

Protein-Rich Chocolate Shake

Prepartion time

5 minutes

INGREDIENTS

- 1 packet Truvia sweetener
- 2 tsp. dark hot chocolate powder
- 1/4 cup cottage cheese, 2%
- 3/4 cup skim milk
- 1/4 tsp vanilla extract
- 4 ice cubes

Instructions

1. Combine all ingredients in a blender and blend until smooth. Enjoy!

Nutrisystem Legal White Chicken Chili

Prepartion time

9 hours

INGREDIENTS

- 12 oz Boneless, Skinless Chicken Breast Cubed
- 1 Can Great Northern Beans
- 3 Cups Fat Free Chicken Broth
- 1 Package of McCormick White Chicken Chili Mix

- 1 Med Onion Chopped

Instructions

1. Combine all ingredients in crock pot set on low. Cook 7 to 9 hours.

Peanut Butter Oatmeal Cookies- Nutrisystem Legal

Prepartion time

27 minutes

INGREDIENTS

- 1 Cup creamy reduced fat penut butter

- 1/2 Cup of oatmeal
- 1/2 Cup of Splenda Brown Sugar Blend
- 1/4 Cup Egg Beaters
- 1 Tblsp Whole Wheat Flour
- 1 tsp cinnamon
- 1 tsp vanilla

Instructions

1. Preheat oven to 350 degrees Makes 12 servings of 2 cookies

2. Mix all ingredients into a medium sized bowl.

3. Mix thorought until well blended.

4. Divide into 24 1" balls.

5. Press long-tined fork into splenda and press into the balls making a cross hatched design.

6. Cook for 12 mins. and move to cooling rack.

7. Store in airtight container.

Easy Whole Wheat Pancakes - Nutrisystem Legal

Prepartion time

20 minutes

INGREDIENTS

- 1/3 cup Hodgson Mill Whole wheat Pancake Mix
- 1 tsp baking powder

- 1 Tbsp Splenda
- 1/4 cup FF milk
- 2 Tbsp egg beaters
- 1/2 tsp vanilla

Instructions

1. Mix flour, baking powder, and Splenda together.

2. Gently stir in milk, egg beaters, and vanilla.

3. Pour onto hot sprayed griddle and cook until golden on each side. Makes

4. Counts as your breakfast entree (add your dairy/protein serving and fruit to complete breakfast).

Easy Cheese burger Pie- Nutrisystem Legal

Prepartion time

45 minutes

INGREDIENTS

- 12 oz 96/4 % lean ground beef
- 1 diced up medium onion
- 1/2 tsp salt or your favorite seasons (I use Cavengers)
- 1 cup FF shredded cheese
- 1/2 cup Heart Smart Bisquick

- 1 cup FF milk
- 1/2 cup egg beaters

Instructions

1. Preheat oven to 400°F
2. Cook lean ground beef with 1 diced up medium onion then add 1/2 tsp salt .
3. Pour into the bottom of a sprayed square baking dish.
4. Top with 1 cup FF shredded cheese
5. MIx Bisquick, milk, and egg beaters.
6. Pour Bisquick mix over it all

7. Bake at 400 degrees for 25 min or until knife comes out clean and crust is brown (took mine about 33 min).

Oatmeal Chocolate Chip Cookies- Nutrisystem Legal

Prepartion time

27 minutes

Ingredients

- 1/2 Cup Dark Chocolate Chips
- 3 tbsp fat free promise spread
- 1 tbsp vegetable oil

- 1 1/2 Cup Instant Oatmeal
- 3 tsp baking powder
- 1/4 Cup of egg beaters
- 1 Cup skim or fat free dry milk powder (do not use greate value)
- 1 tsp Vanillia Extract
- 1/2 Cup Whole Wheat Flour
- 3 tbsp Slenda brown sugar blend
- Non stick butter spray

Instructions

1. Pre heat oven to 325. Spray 2 cookie sheets with butter flavored Crisco

2. Mix dry fat milk powder with1/2 cup tepid water and set aside.

3. Use medium size bowl to mix together flour, oatmeal, baking powder, and salt. Set aside.

4. Using a wisk, in a large bowl cream promise and brown sugar. Add oil and mix.

5. Wisk in eggs. Then wisk in vanillia, followed by milk mixture and egg beaters.

6. Use spoon to mix in flour mixture.

7. Stir in chocolate chips.

8. This dough is not very dense as in normal cookies. Do not worry. Drop by tablespoon to make 20 cookies.

9. Spread any unused dough in the bowl evenly between the cookies.

10. I normally spray the tops of each cookie very well with butter spray. Then I spray my fingers with the butter spray

11. mash the cookies into a larger shape.

12. Cool on wire rack and serve.

13. When the left over cookies are cool , put 2 cookies in a snack bag and freeze to use at another time. They will keep up to 2 months.

Nutri System Leagal - Crab Cakes

Prepartion time

30 minutes

INGREDIENTS

- 1/4 Cup finely chopped onion
- 2 Tablespoons fresh parsley
- 3 Tablespoons light Mayo
- 2 Teaspoons of Dijon Mustard
- 3/4 Teaspoon Worcestershire sause
- 1 LBS lump crabmeat, drain and shell pieces emoved
- 1 1/2 Cups pancko (Japanese breadcrumbs) Divided
- 1 Tablespoon olive oil divided
- 1 Large Jalapeno diced Into small Pieces (Optional)
- Cooking Spray

Instructions

1. Combine first 7 ingredients in medium bowl. Gently fold in crab meat. Gently sir in 3/4 cup panko. Cover and chill 30 minutes.

2. Divide Crab mixture into 8 equal portions (about 1/2 cup each);shape each into a 3/4 inch thick patty.

3. Place remaining panko in a shallow bowl. Dredge 1 patty in panko. Repeat with remaining patties and panko.

4. Heat 1 1/2 seaspons oil in medium nonstick skillet over medium heat. Coat both sidedes of crab cake with cooking spray.

5. Add 4 crab cakes to pan; cook 7 minutes. Carefully turn over;cook 7 minutes or until golden.

6. Repeat Procedure with remaining 1 1/2 , cooking spray, and remaining 4 crab cakes.

Chicken and Broccoli-Parmesan Pasta

Prepartion time

40 minutes

Ingredients

- 2 1/2 C whole wheat penne pasta or rotini
- 3 C broccoli, cut into florets (or substitute frozen, chopped broccoli)
- 1 lb skinless, boneless chicken breast, cut into bite-sized pieces
- 1 tsp adobo seasoning

- 1 clove garlic, minced
- 1/4 C fat-free cream cheese, softened and cut into small pieces
- 2 Tbsp shaved Parmesan cheese

Instructions

1. To make adobo seasoning, if not readily available, combine 1 teaspoon each: onion powder, cumin, cayenne pepper, oregano, black pepper, and garlic powder. You will only need 1 tsp of the mixture for this recipe. Store the remainder in a dry container.

2. Cook pasta according to package directions.

3. Add broccoli for the last 5 minutes of cooking time. Drain well.

4. Meanwhile, combine chicken pieces and adobo seasoning, coating chicken well. Prepare a large skillet with cooking spray.

5. Heat skillet to medium.

6. Add garlic and stir for about 30 seconds.

7. Add chicken pieces.

8. Cook chicken thoroughly, stirring occasionally, about 3 to 5 minutes.

9. Add pasta and broccoli to the chicken skillet.

10. Stir in cream cheese. Cook over low heat until cream cheese has melted and coated the mixture.

11. To serve, sprinkle with parmesan cheese.

Nutri System Legal Sally's Individual Meat Loaves

Prepartion time

1 hour

INGREDIENTS

- 12oz Lean hambuger meat
- 3 Slices of reduced calorie wheat bread (I use

White

- Wheat) torn into small pieces.
- 1 Small onion chopped
- 1/4 tsp dry mustard

- 1 tsp salt
- 1 Tbsp Horseradish
- 1 tsp worchestershire sause
- 1/4 Cup of eggbeaters
- 1/4 Cup of fat free milk
- 2 Tbsp Catsup

Instructions

1. Spray 9" X 9" baking pan with pam.

2. Preheat oven to 400.

3. In a medium bowl combine hambuger, bread, onion, dry mustard, and salt.

4. Add Horseradish, worchestershire, eggbeaters, and milk until blended well.

5. Divide mixture into 3 equal balls.

6. Shape balls into oval loaf shape and place in prepared pan.

7. Bake for 20 minutes.

8. Squeeze catsup in a line in the middle of each meat loaf.

9. Bake for additional 10 minutes.

10. If baking frozen meat loafs cook for 30 minutes and spread on catsup.

11. Bake additional 10 minutes.

Chicken Parmesan Pasta

Prepartion time

35 minutes

INGREDIENTS

- Parmesan Cheese, grated, 2 tbsp
- Olive Oil, 1 tbsp
- Chicken Breast (cooked), no skin, 1.50 lb ready-to-cook chicken)
- Garlic, 2 clove
- Onions, raw, 0.25 cup, chopped
- Green Peppers (bell peppers), 0.25 cup, chopped Crushed Tomatoes, 1/2 Lg Can
- Spinach, frozen, 1 cup
- Barilla - White Fiber Mini Penne Pasta, 6 oz (half box)

Instructions

1. Put the olive oil in a large pan.

2. Saute onions, garlic, peppers and chicken together until chicken is cooked through.

3. While you are doing that, get a pot of boiling water ready for the pasta.

4. Once chicken is done, add the tomatoes to the pan with the parmesan cheese. boil the pasta as directed on the box.

5. Simmer the pan of chicken & sauce very low.

6. When the pasta is done, drain and add it to the pan of sauce.

7. Add in the spinach and mix well.

8. Simer over low heat for about 5 minutes and then sprinkle with a bit of parsley and a little shredded mozzarella as garnish. Enjoy!

Roasted Potatoes, Carrorts, and Green Onions

Prepartion time

50 minutes

INGREDIENTS

- 5 Med to small red skin potatoes, cut into 1/4"wedges
- 6-10 Green onions cut into 2 inch sections and halfed

- 3 Large Carrots cut into match sticks size pieces
- Cavengers Seasoning
- Butter flavored cooking spray

Instructions

1. Pre Heat oven to 450
2. Spray bottom of 9x13 baking pan with cooking spray.
3. Place potatoe wedges in bottom of pan spray again with cooking spray and sprinkle cavengers to taste (or use your favorite seasoning).
4. Next, layer carrots on top of potates, spray with cooking spray and seasoning.

5. Top with green onions and repeat with cooking spray and seasoning.

6. Turn mixture every 10 minutes and spray with cooking spray.

7. Potatoes should be brown and crispy.Enjoy

Black beans, corn, and rice

Prepartion time

1 hour 5 minutes

INGREDIENTS

- 4 cups cooked rice
- 1 (15 ounce) can black beans, rinsed and drained

- 1 (15 ounce) can corn, drained
- 2 fresh tomatoes, diced
- 1/2 cup red onions, chopped
- 1/2 cup cilantro, chopped
- 2 tablespoons fresh lime juice
- 1 tablespoon olive oil
- 1/2 teaspoon salt
- 1/4 teaspoon fresh ground pepper
- 2 dashes hot sauce

Instructions

1. Cook rice according to instructions

2. In a medium bowl, combine black beans, corn, tomatoes, onion, cilantro, jalapeno, lime juice, oil, salt, pepper and hot sauce.

3. To serve, Place a scoop of hot rice in a bowl or on a plate, top with a generous scoop of the black bean mixture.

4. Stir together before eating.

Veggie Egg Scramble

Prepartion time

10 minutes

INGREDIENTS

- Non-Stick Olive Oil Cooking Spray

- 2 Egg whites
- 1 Strip Chopped Green Bell Pepper
- 1 Strip Chopped Red Bell Pepper
- 1 Strip Chopped Yellow Bell Pepper
- 1 Medium Slice Chopped Onion
- 1 tbsp Diced Tomatoes
- 10 Leaves Chopped Fresh Spinach
- 1 Dash Black Pepper

Instructions

1. Spray pan with Non-Stick Olive Oil Cooking Spray.

2. Saute onions and peppers.

3. Have eggs pre-cracked or measured.

4. Add in spinach, tomato, and black pepper.

5. Add in egg and stir.

6. Enjoy!

Hearty Beef & Vegetable Stew

Prepartion time

1 hour

Ingredients:

- 1 lb - Lein Stew Beef (or Chuck), cubed
- 1 - Onion, small - course chop
- 1 - Garlic, 1 clove - minced

- 1 tbsp - *Extra Light Olive Oil
- 1 pkg - Baby Carrots - coarse chop
- 12 small - New Potatoes (or small Red) - quartered
- 1/2 lb - Green Beans - coarse chop
- 1 - 14.5 oz Canned Tomatoes (or stewed)
- 4 tsp - Better Than Beef Boullion
- 1/4 cup - Corn Starch
- Pepper to taste

Instructions

1. Saute garlic and onions in EVOO (about 1 minute); add beef cubes and brown.

2. Add 2.5 quarts (10 cups) of water, the carrotts and potatoes, and beef boullion. Bring to boil, stir, then cover 10-15 minutes.

3. Add canned tomatoes and green beans.

4. Can add corn starch to thicken. Season with pepper. Salt is optional as Beef Boullion can be salty. (Another 1 tsp can be added, to taste).

Baked Chicken Egg Rolls

Prepartion time

55 minutes

INGREDIENTS

- 3 C bagged coleslaw mix, divided

- 1/4 C sliced water chestnuts (about 10 slices)
- 1/4 C green onions
- 2 tea canola oil
- 1 T minced ginger
- 4 cloves garlic, minced
- 1/4 C grated onion
- 1lb ground chicken (boneless, skinless chicken breast, ground)
- 1/4 t kosher salt
- 2 tea low sodium soy sauce
- 1 package egg roll wrappers
- Non-Stick Cooking Spray

Instructions

1. Preheat oven to 425 Degrees.

2. Spray a baking sheet with non-stick cooking spray. Set aside.

3. In a food processor, combine 1 C of the bagged coleslaw, water chestnuts, and green onions.

4. Pulse about 12 times or until ground into small pieces. Set aside.

5. Mince garlic cloves and ginger.

6. Grate onion until you have 1/4 C.

7. In an extra large skillet on the stove top heat canola oil.

8. Leave temperature at medium-high. Add the minced ginger, minced garlic, and grated onion.

9. Saute for 2-3 minutes or until tender. Add the ground chicken and kosher salt.

10. Cook until chicken is no longer pink.

11. Add cabbage mixture to skillet along with the 2 C additional coleslaw mix. Saute for 2 minutes and then add soy sauce.

12. Cook one minute longer and then remove from heat.

13. Place 3-4 T filling in each egg roll wrapper and roll to seal.

14. Place on baking sheet and spray the tops lightly with cooking spray.

15. Bake in preheated oven for 20-25 minutes or until browned on the edges. (If under-baked, egg rolls will be chewy!)

16. Let cool for 5-10 minutes before serving.

Slow Cooker Quinoa Carrot Breakfast Bowl

Prepartion time

3 hours 40 minutes

Ingredients

- 1 cup uncooked quinoa
- 3 cups unsweetened almond milk with added protein
- 1 small zucchini, grated
- 2 carrots, grated

- 3 Tbsp. shredded unsweetened coconut
- 1 Tbsp. chia seeds
- ¼ tsp. ground nutmeg
- 2 tsp. ground cinnamon
- ¼ tsp. salt
- 1 tsp. vanilla extract
- 3-4 stevia packets
- 1 Tbsp. chopped walnuts, for topping

Instructions

1. Wash, dry and grate zucchini. Put shredded zucchini in a clean dishtowel and squeeze out the excess liquid.

2. Wash, dry and grate carrots.

3. Add all ingredients, except walnuts, to a 5 to 6-quart slow cooker.

4. Stir contents of slow cooker with a large spoon until combined.

5. Cover and cook on low for 3 hours stirring occasionally.

6. To serve, top with 1 Tbsp. chopped walnuts.

Vegetable Lasagna Bake

Prepartion time

1 hour 10 minutes

Ingredients

- 6 lasagna noodles

- 2 cups frozen spinach, thawed and drained
- 2 cups butternut squash
- 1 tomato, sliced
- 2 cups low fat cottage cheese or ricotta cheese
- 2 eggs
- 2 tsp. Italian seasoning
- 2 cups shredded mozzarella cheese, low fat
- Zero calorie cooking spray

Instructions

1. Preheat oven to 350 F. Lightly coat a small casserole dish or loaf pan with cooking spray

2. Cook lasagna noodles according to package directions

3. Fill a medium pot with water and bring to boil. Add butternut squash and cook until soft. Drain then mash with a fork

4. Combine cottage/ricotta cheese, eggs and Italian seasoning

Lasagna Assembly:

1. Place 2 lasagna noodles on bottom of casserole dish. Spread ½ of mashed butternut squash on the noodles. Top with ½ of the spinach and tomato. Add 1/3 of the cottage/ricotta cheese mixture and mozzarella cheese. Repeat.

2. Top with last two lasagna noodles, then spread the rest of the cottage/ricotta cheese mixture and mozzarella.

3. Cover with foil and bake for 35 minutes.

4. Remove cover and bake for an additional 10 minutes.

Slow Cooker Chicken Gumbo

Prepartion time

6 hours

Ingredients

- 1 c up low sodium chicken broth
- 2, 14.5 oz. cans of diced fire roasted tomatoes, undrained
- 16 oz. chicken breast, cut into cubes

- 1 large onion, chopped
- 1 large green bell pepper, chopped
- 4 stalks of celery, chopped
- 1.5 cups of corn (fresh or frozen)
- 1.5 Tbsp. creole seasoning
- ¼ tsp. ground black pepper
- ¼ tsp. cayenne pepper
- 1.5 cups brown rice, cooked

Instructions

1. Cut chicken into 1-inch cubes.

2. Wash and chop onion, green bell pepper, and celery.

3. Add chicken broth, tomatoes, chicken, onion, green bell pepper, celery and corn to a 5 to 6-quart slow cooker. Then, add in creole seasoning, black pepper, and cayenne pepper.

4. Stir contents of slow cooker with a large spoon until combined.

5. Cover and cook on low for 5-6 hours stirring occasionally.

6. Stir well before serving. Serve over cooked brown rice.

Sheet Pan Shrimp Fajitas

Prepartion time

10 minutes

Ingredients

- 1 1/2 lbs. of shrimp, peeled and deveined
- 1 yellow bell pepper, sliced thin
- 1 red bell pepper, sliced thin
- 1 orange bell pepper, sliced thin
- 1 small red onion, sliced thin
- 1 1/2 Tbsp. of extra virgin olive oil
- 1 tsp. of kosher salt
- freshly ground pepper

- 2 tsp. chili powder
- 1/2 tsp. garlic powder
- 1/2 tsp. onion powder
- 1/2 tsp. of ground cumin
- 1/2 teaspoon of smoked paprika
- lime
- fresh cilantro for garnish
- 6 whole wheat tortilla, warmed

Instructions

1. Preheat oven to 450 F and spray baking sheet with zero-calorie nonstick cooking spray.

2. Combine shrimp, onion, bell pepper, olive oil and dry spices in a large bowl.

3. Pour contents across baking sheet and spread evenly.

4. Cook for about 8 minutes. Switch oven to broil and cook for 2 more minutes or until the shrimp is fully cooked.

5. Remove baking sheet, add lime juice and season with fresh cilantro. Serve with warmed, whole wheat tortilla.

Stuffed Acorn Squash

Preparation time

50 minutes

Ingredients:

- 1 acorn squash
- 1 cup cooked quinoa
- ½ cup pomegranate seeds (or 1/4 cup dried cranberries)
- 8 Tbsp. crushed walnuts
- 1 tsp. coriander
- Dried parsley
- Zero-calorie cooking spray

Instructions

1. Preheat oven to 400 F.

2. Slice acorn squash into 4 slices and remove the seeds (If too hard, poke holes and microwave for 4 minutes to allow it to soften).

3. Place on an aluminum-lined baking sheet and spray lightly with cooking spray.

4. Bake for 35-40 minutes or until soft.

5. Mix together quinoa, walnuts, pomegranate, and coriander.

6. Fill each squash with quinoa mixture and sprinkle dried parsley on top.

Meat & Potato Casserole

Prepartion time

1 hour 6 minutes

Ingredients:

- 9 oz. lean ground turkey

- 1 small onion, chopped
- 3 medium potatoes, peeled
- 1 ½ cups shredded carrot
- 2 large whole eggs
- 2 large egg whites
- ¼ cup low sodium chicken broth
- 2 Tbsp. whole wheat flour
- 1 ½ tsp. black pepper
- Zero calorie cooking spray

Instructions

1. Preheat oven to 400 °F.

2. Add turkey to a greased pan on medium-high heat and cook, until it is no longer pink.

3. Grate potatoes in a food processor.

4. Put grated potatoes in a colander and squeeze excess water out.

5. In a mixing bowl, combine all ingredients.

6. Pour in a greased 8 x 8 baking dish.

7. Spray top of it with cooking spray.

8. Bake for 20 minutes.

9. Lower heat to 325 °F and bake for another 30-40 minutes.

Marinated Greek Chicken Skewers

Prepartion time

45 minutes

Ingredients:

- 1 lb. boneless, skinless chicken breast, cut into 1-inch pieces
- 2 Tbsp. extra virgin olive oil, divided
- 4 garlic cloves, crushed
- 1-2 tsp. dried oregano
- 1 tsp. salt
- 1 tsp. ground black pepper

- 2 Tbsp. freshly squeezed lemon juice
- 1/2 red onion, quartered
- 1 green bell pepper, cut into 1-inch pieces
- 1 red bell pepper, cut into 1-inch pieces
- Skewers

Instructions

1. Spray chicken with cooking spray then toss in garlic, oregano, salt and pepper and let marinade for 30 minutes.

2. In a small bowl, whisk together remaining olive oil and lemon juice. Set aside.

3. Preheat indoor grill pan to medium-high heat.

4. Thread skewers, alternating chicken and vegetables.

5. Grill, turning and drizzling with sauce mixture, until chicken is cooked through.

Sweet Potato Noodle Bowl with Creamy Almond Butter Sauce

Prepartion time

20 minutes

Ingredients:

- Noodle Bowl
- 6 oz. cooked shrimp

- 2 cups sweet potato, spiralized or peeled into thin strips
- 2 tsp. olive oil
- 2 cups raw spinach
- Cayenne pepper, to taste
- Black pepper, to taste

Almond Butter Sauce

- 2 Tbsp. almond butter
- 1/3 cup chicken broth, low sodium
- 1 tsp. light soy sauce
- ½ tsp. garlic powder

Instructions

1. In a large sauté pan, heat olive oil over medium heat.

2. Add sweet potatoes to pan and toss frequently.

3. In the meantime, make the almond butter sauce by combining all ingredients in a small pot.

4. Heat sauce and stir, until it simmers and a creamy sauce forms.

5. Pour almond butter sauce over sweet potato noodles.

6. Cook until sweet potatoes are soft.

7. Stir in spinach, shrimp, cayenne pepper, black pepper and serve.

www.ingramcontent.com/pod-product-compliance
Ingram Content Group UK Ltd.
Pitfield, Milton Keynes, MK11 3LW, UK
UKHW022006190726
13853UKWH00004B/1761